The Ultimate Dash Diet Cookbook

50+ Fast and Yummy Ideas for Your Everyday Meals

Eleonore Barlow

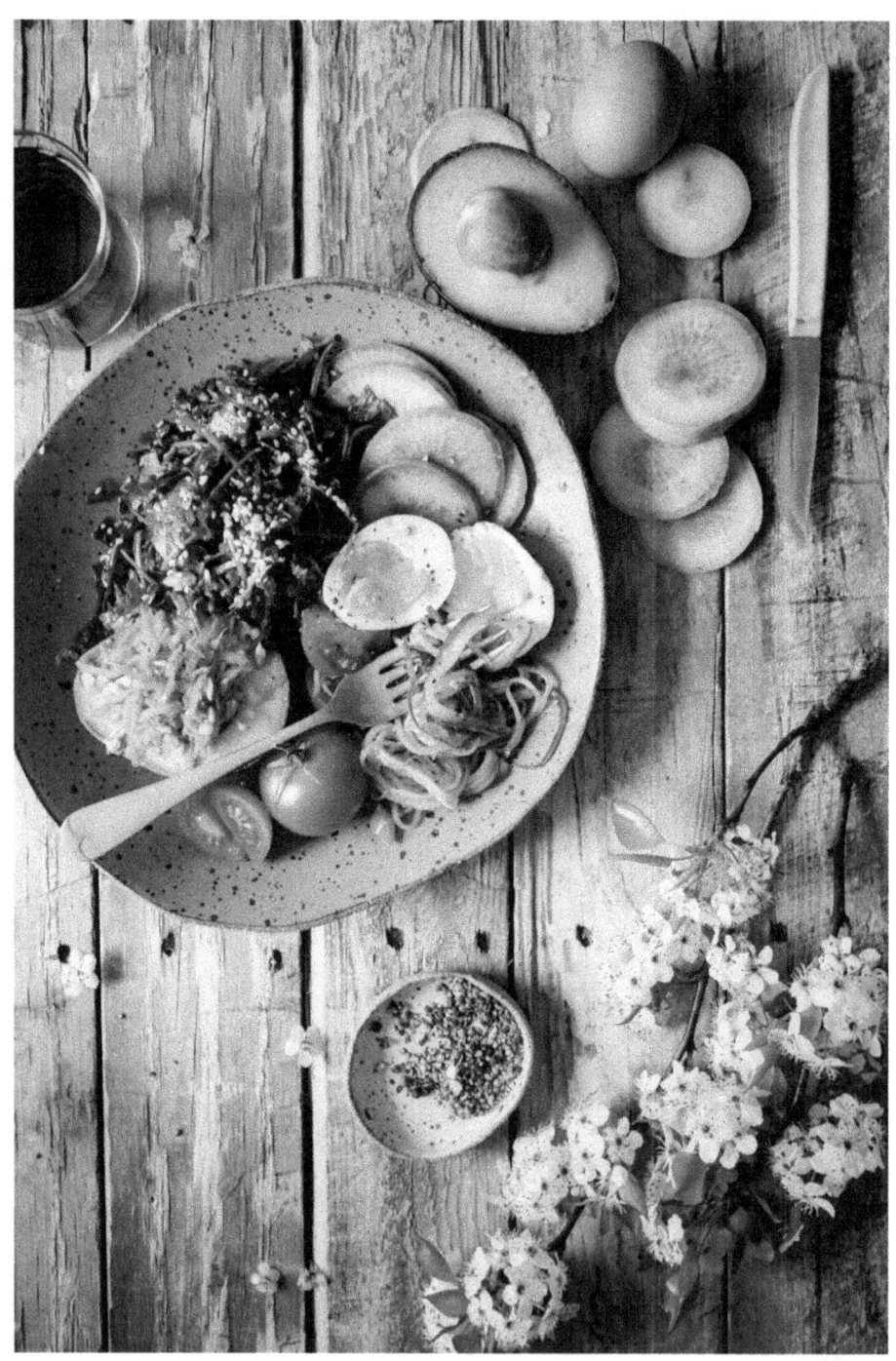

© Copyright 2021 - All rights reserved.

The content contained within this book may not be reproduced, duplicated or transmitted without direct written permission from the author or the publisher.
Under no circumstances will any blame or legal responsibility be held against the publisher, or author, for any damages, reparation, or monetary loss due to the information contained within this book. Either directly or indirectly.

Legal Notice:
This book is copyright protected. This book is only for personal use. You cannot amend, distribute, sell, use, quote or paraphrase any part, or the content within this book, without the consent of the author or publisher.

Disclaimer Notice:
Please note the information contained within this document is for educational and entertainment purposes only. All effort has been executed to present accurate, up to date, and reliable, complete information. No warranties of any kind are declared or implied. Readers acknowledge that the author is not engaging in the rendering of legal, financial, medical or professional advice. The content within this book has been derived from various sources. Please consult a licensed professional before attempting any techniques outlined in this book.
By reading this document, the reader agrees that under no circumstances is the author responsible for any losses, direct or indirect, which are incurred as a result of the use of information contained within this document, including, but not limited to, — errors, omissions, or inaccuracies.

Table of Contents

CHIA PORRIDGE 6
MOUTHWATERING CHICKEN PORRIDGE 8
SIMPLE BLUEBERRY OATMEAL 10
THE DECISIVE APPLE "PORRIDGE" 12
THE UNIQUE SMOOTHIE BOWL 14
CINNAMON AND COCONUT PORRIDGE 16
MORNING PORRIDGE 18
TANTALIZING CAULIFLOWER AND DILL MASH 20
SECRET ASIAN GREEN BEANS 22
EXCELLENT ACORN MIX 24
CRUNCHY ALMOND CHOCOLATE BARS 26
LETTUCE AND CHICKEN PLATTER 29
CHIPOTLE LETTUCE CHICKEN 31
BALSAMIC CHICKEN AND VEGETABLES 34
CREAM DREDGED CORN PLATTER 36
EXUBERANT SWEET POTATOES 38
LEEK AND CAULIFLOWER SOUP 40
DREAMY ZUCCHINI BOWL 42
COLD CRAB AND WATERMELON SOUP 44
PALEO LEMON AND GARLIC SOUP 46
BRUSSELS SOUP 48
SPRING SOUP AND POACHED EGG 50
LOBSTER BISQUE 52
TOMATO BISQUE 54
CHIPOTLE CHICKEN CHOWDER 56
CINNAMON SALMON 58

SCALLOP AND STRAWBERRY MIX	60
SALMON AND ORANGE DISH	62
MESMERIZING COCONUT HADDOCK	64
ASPARAGUS AND LEMON SALMON DISH	66
LAMB CURRY WITH TOMATOES AND SPINACH	68
POMEGRANATE-MARINATED LEG OF LAMB	70
BEEF FAJITAS WITH PEPPERS	72
PORK MEDALLIONS WITH HERBS DE PROVENCE	75
RAVAGING BLUEBERRY MUFFIN	77
THE COCONUT LOAF	79
FRESH FIGS WITH WALNUTS AND RICOTTA	81
AUTHENTIC MEDJOOL DATE TRUFFLES	83
TASTY MEDITERRANEAN PEANUT ALMOND BUTTER POPCORNS	85
JUST A MINUTE WORTH MUFFIN	87
HEARTY ALMOND BREAD	89
REFRESHING MANGO AND PEAR SMOOTHIE	91
COCONUT AND HAZELNUT CHILLED GLASS	93
THE MOCHA SHAKE	94
CINNAMON CHILLER	95
HEARTY ALKALINE STRAWBERRY SUMMER DELUXE	97
MESMERIZING BRUSSELS AND PISTACHIOS	99
BRUSSELS'S FEVER	101
HEARTY GARLIC AND KALE PLATTER	103
ACORN SQUASH WITH MANGO CHUTNEY	105

Chia Porridge

Serving: 2

Prep Time: 10 minutes

Cook Time: 5-10 minutes

Ingredients:

1 tablespoon chia seeds

1 tablespoon ground flaxseed

1/3 cup coconut cream

½ cup water

1 teaspoon vanilla extract

1 tablespoon almond butter

How To:

1. Add chia seeds, coconut milk, flaxseed, water and vanilla to a little pot.

2. Stir and let it sit for five minutes.

3. Add almond butter and place pot over low heat.

4. Keep stirring as almond butter melts.

5. Once the porridge is hot/not boiling, pour into bowl.

6. Enjoy!

7. Add a couple of berries or a touch of cream for extra flavor.

Nutrition (Per Serving)

Calories: 410

Fat: 38g

Carbohydrates: 10g

Protein: 6g

Mouthwatering Chicken Porridge

Serving: 4

Prep Time: 1 hour

Cook Time: 10-20 minutes

Ingredients:

1 cup jasmine rice

1 pound steamed/cooked chicken legs

5 cups chicken broth

4 cups water

1 ½ cups fresh ginger

Green onions

Toasted cashew nuts

How To:

1. Place the rice in your fridge and permit it to relax 1 hour before cooking.

2. Take the rice out and add it to your Instant Pot.

3. Pour in chicken stock and water.

4. Lock the lid and cook on PORRIDGE mode, using the default settings and parameters.

5. Release the pressure naturally over 10 minutes.

6. Open the lid.

7. Remove the meat from the chicken legs and add the meat to your soup.

8. Stir overflow Sauté mode.

9. Season with a touch of flavored vinegar and luxuriate in with a garnish of nuts and onion.

Nutrition (Per Serving)

Calories: 206

Fat: 8g

Carbohydrates: 8g

Protein: 23g

Simple Blueberry Oatmeal

Serving: 4

Prep Time: 10 minutes

Cooking Time: 8 hours

Ingredients:

1 cup blueberries

1 cup steel-cut oats1 cup coconut milk

2 tablespoons agave nectar

½ teaspoon vanilla extract Coconut flakes, garnish

How To:

1. Grease Slow Cooker with cooking spray.
2. Add oats, milk, nectar, blueberries, and vanilla.
3. Toss well.
4. Place lid and cook on LOW for 8 hours.
5. Divide between serving bowls and serve.
6. Enjoy!

Nutrition (Per Serving)

Calories: 202

Fat: 6g

Carbohydrates: 12g

Protein: 6g

The Decisive Apple "Porridge"

Serving: 2

Prep Time: 10 minutes

Cook Time: 5 minutes

Ingredients:

1 large apple, peeled, cored and grated

1 cup unsweetened almond milk

1 ½ tablespoons sunflower seeds

1/8 cup fresh blueberries

¼ teaspoon fresh vanilla bean extract

How To:

1. Take an outsized pan and add sunflower seeds, vanilla, almond milk, apples, and stir.

2. Place over medium-low heat.

3. Cook for five minutes, ensuring to stay the mixture stirring.

4. Transfer to a serving bowl.

5. Serve and enjoy!

Nutrition (Per Serving)

Calories: 123

Fat: 1.3g

Carbohydrates:23g

Protein: 4g

The Unique Smoothie Bowl

Serving: 2

Prep Time: 10 minutes

Cook Time: Nil

Ingredients:

2 cups baby spinach leaves

1 cup coconut almond milk

¼ cup low fat cream

2 tablespoons flaxseed oil

2 tablespoons chia seeds

2 tablespoons walnuts, roughly chopped A handful of fresh berries

How To:

1. Add spinach leaves, coconut almond milk, cream and linseed oil to a blender.

2. Blitz until smooth.

3. Pour smoothie into serving bowls.

4. Sprinkle chia seeds, berries, walnuts on top.

5. Serve and enjoy!

Nutrition (Per Serving)

Calories: 380

Fat: 36g

Carbohydrates: 12g

Protein: 5g

Cinnamon and Coconut Porridge

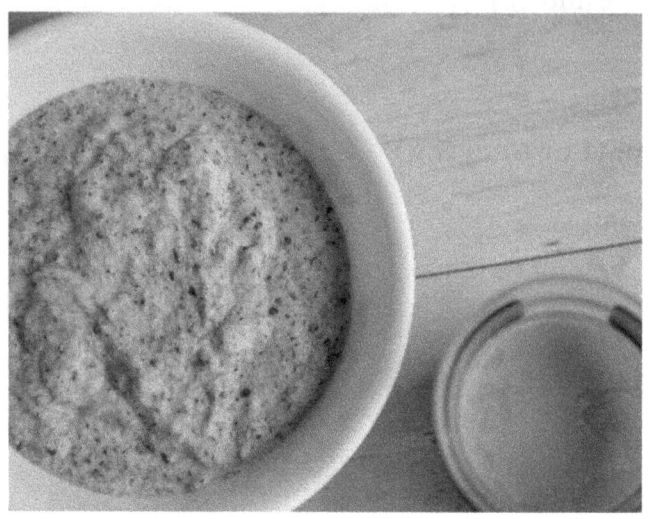

Serving: 4

Prep Time: 5 minutes

Cook Time: 5 minutes

Ingredients:

2 cups water

1 cup coconut cream

½ cup unsweetened dried coconut, shredded 2 tablespoons flaxseed meal 1 tablespoon almond butter

1 ½ teaspoons stevia

1 teaspoon cinnamon

Toppings as blueberries

How To:

1. Add the listed ingredients to a little pot, mix well.

2. Transfer pot to stove and place over medium-low heat.

3. bring back mix to a slow boil.

4. Stir well and take away from the warmth.

5. Divide the combination into equal servings and allow them to sit for 10 minutes.

6. Top together with your desired toppings and enjoy!

Nutrition (Per Serving)

Calories: 171

Fat: 16g

Carbohydrates: 6g

Protein: 2g

Morning Porridge

Serving: 2

Prep Time: 15 minutes

Cook Time: Nil

Ingredients:

2 tablespoons coconut flour

2 tablespoons vanilla protein powder

3 tablespoons Golden Flaxseed meal

1 ½ cups almond milk, unsweetened Powdered erythritol

How To:

1. Take a bowl and blend in flaxseed meal, protein powder, coconut flour and blend well.
2. Add mix to the saucepan (place over medium heat).
3. Add almond milk and stir, let the mixture thicken.
4. Add your required amount of sweetener and serve.
5. Enjoy!

Nutrition (Per Serving)

Calories: 259

Fat: 13g

Carbohydrates: 5g

Protein: 16g

Tantalizing Cauliflower and Dill Mash

Serving: 6

Prep Time: 10 minutes

Cooking Time: 6 hours

Ingredients:

1 cauliflower head, florets separated

1/3 cup dill, chopped

6 garlic cloves

2 tablespoons olive oil

Pinch of black pepper

How To:

1. Add cauliflower to Slow Cooker.

2. Add dill, garlic and water to hide them. 3. Place lid and cook on HIGH for five hours.

3. Drain the flowers.

4. Season with pepper and add oil, mash using potato masher.

5. Whisk and serve.

6. Enjoy!

Nutrition (Per Serving)

Calories: 207

Fat: 4g

Carbohydrates: 14g

Protein: 3g

Secret Asian Green Beans

Serving: 10

Prep Time: 10 minutes

Cooking Time: 2 hours

Ingredients:

16 cups green beans, halved

3 tablespoons olive oil

¼ cup tomato sauce, salt-free

½ cup coconut sugar

¾ teaspoon low sodium soy sauce

Pinch of pepper

How To:

1. Add green beans, coconut sugar, pepper spaghetti sauce, soy sauce, oil to your Slow Cooker.

2. Stir well.

3. Place lid and cook on LOW for 3 hours.

4. Divide between serving platters and serve.

5. Enjoy!

Nutrition (Per Serving)

Calories: 200

Fat: 4g

Carbohydrates: 12g

Protein: 3g

Excellent Acorn Mix

Serving: 10

Prep Time: 10 minutes

Cooking Time: 7 hours

Ingredients:

2 acorn squash, peeled and cut into wedges

16 ounces cranberry sauce, unsweetened

¼ teaspoon cinnamon powder Pepper to taste

How To:

1. Add acorn wedges to your Slow Cooker.
2. Add condiment, cinnamon, raisins and pepper.
3. Stir.
4. Place lid and cook on LOW for 7 hours.
5. Serve and enjoy!

Nutrition (Per Serving)

Calories: 200

Fat: 3g

Carbohydrates: 15g

Protein: 2g

Crunchy Almond Chocolate Bars

Serving: 12

Prep Time: 10 minutes

Cooking Time: 2 hours 30 minutes

Ingredients:

1 egg white

¼ cup coconut oil, melted

1 cup coconut sugar

½ teaspoon vanilla extract

1 teaspoon baking powder

1 ½ cups almond meal

½ cup dark chocolate chips

How To:

1.   Take a bowl and add sugar, oil, vanilla, egg white, almond flour, leaven and blend it well.

2.   Fold in chocolate chips and stir.

3. Line Slow Cooker with parchment paper.

4. Grease.

5. Add the cookie mix and continue bottom.

6. Place lid and cook on LOW for two hours half-hour .

7. Take cooking utensil out and let it cool.

8. Cut in bars and enjoy!

Nutrition (Per Serving)

Calories: 200

Fat: 2g

Carbohydrates: 13g

Protein: 6g

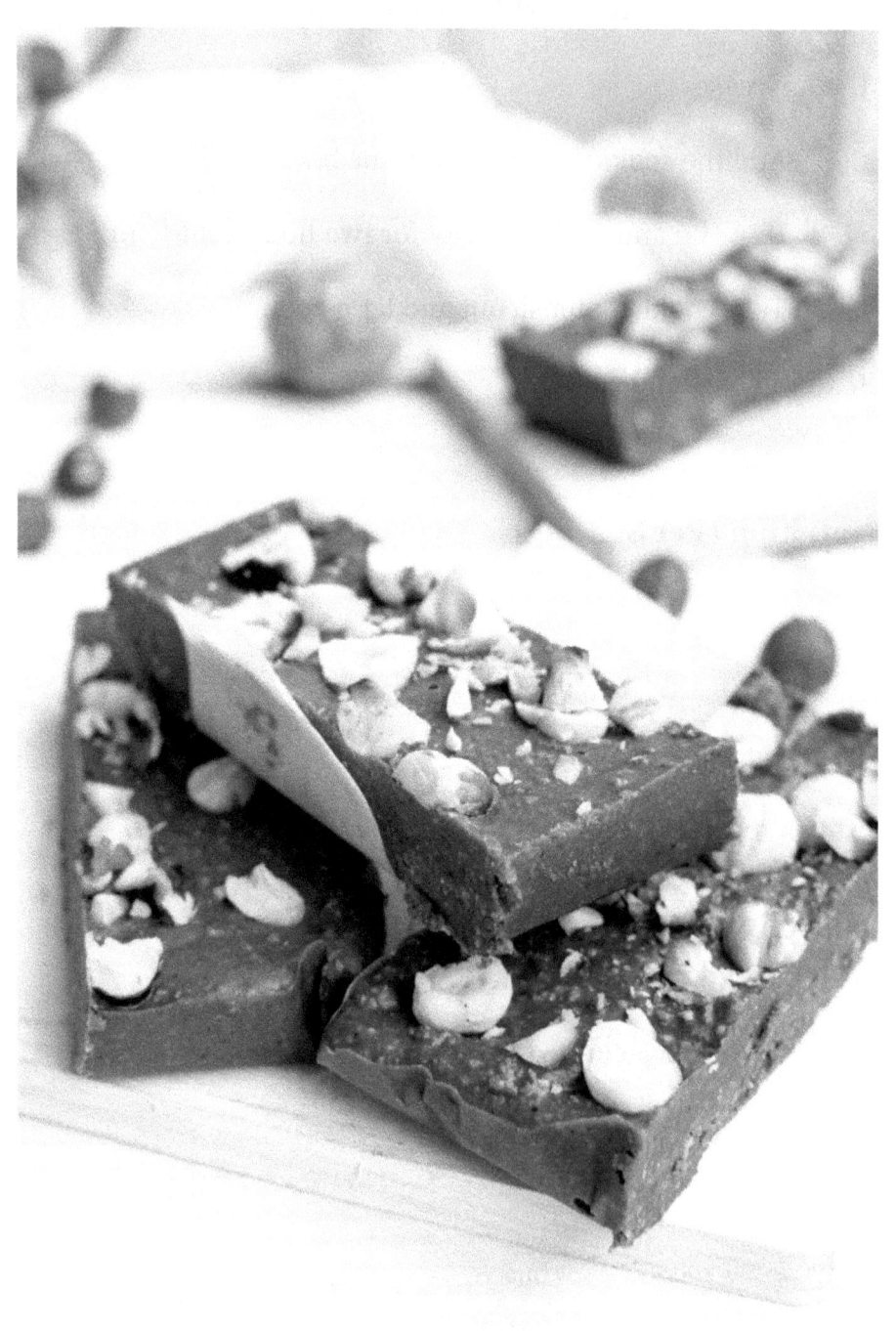

Lettuce and Chicken Platter

Serving: 6

Prep Time: 10 minutes

Cook Time: nil

Ingredients:

2 cups chicken, cooked and coarsely chopped ½ head ice berg lettuce, sliced and chopped 1 celery rib, chopped

1 medium apple, cut

½ red bell pepper, deseeded and chopped 6-7 green olives, pitted and halved 1 red onion, chopped

For dressing

1 tablespoon raw honey

2 tablespoons lemon juice

Salt and pepper to taste

How To:

1. Cut the vegetables and transfer them to your Salad Bowl.
2. Add olives.

3. Chop the cooked chicken and transfer to your Salad bowl.

4. Prepare dressing by mixing the ingredients listed under Dressing.

5. Pour the dressing into the Salad bowl.

6. Toss and enjoy!

Nutrition (Per Serving)

Calories: 296

Fat: 21g

Carbohydrates: 9g

Protein: 18g

Chipotle Lettuce Chicken

Serving: 6

Prep Time: 10 minutes

Cook Time: 25 minutes

Ingredients:

1-pound chicken breast, cut into strips

Splash of olive oil

1 red onion, finely sliced

14 ounces tomatoes

1 teaspoon chipotle, chopped

½ teaspoon cumin

Lettuce as needed

Fresh coriander leaves

Jalapeno chilies, sliced

Fresh tomato slices for garnish

Lime wedges

How To:

1. Take a non-stick frypan and place it over medium heat.

2. Add oil and warmth it up.

3. Add chicken and cook until brown.

4. Keep the chicken on the side.

5. Add tomatoes, sugar, chipotle, cumin to an equivalent pan and simmer for 25 minutes until you've got a pleasant sauce.

6. Add chicken into the sauce and cook for five minutes.

7. Transfer the combination to a different place.

8. Use lettuce wraps to require some of the mixture and serve with a squeeze of lemon.

9. Enjoy!

Nutrition (Per Serving)

Calories: 332

Fat: 15g

Carbohydrates: 13g

Protein: 34g

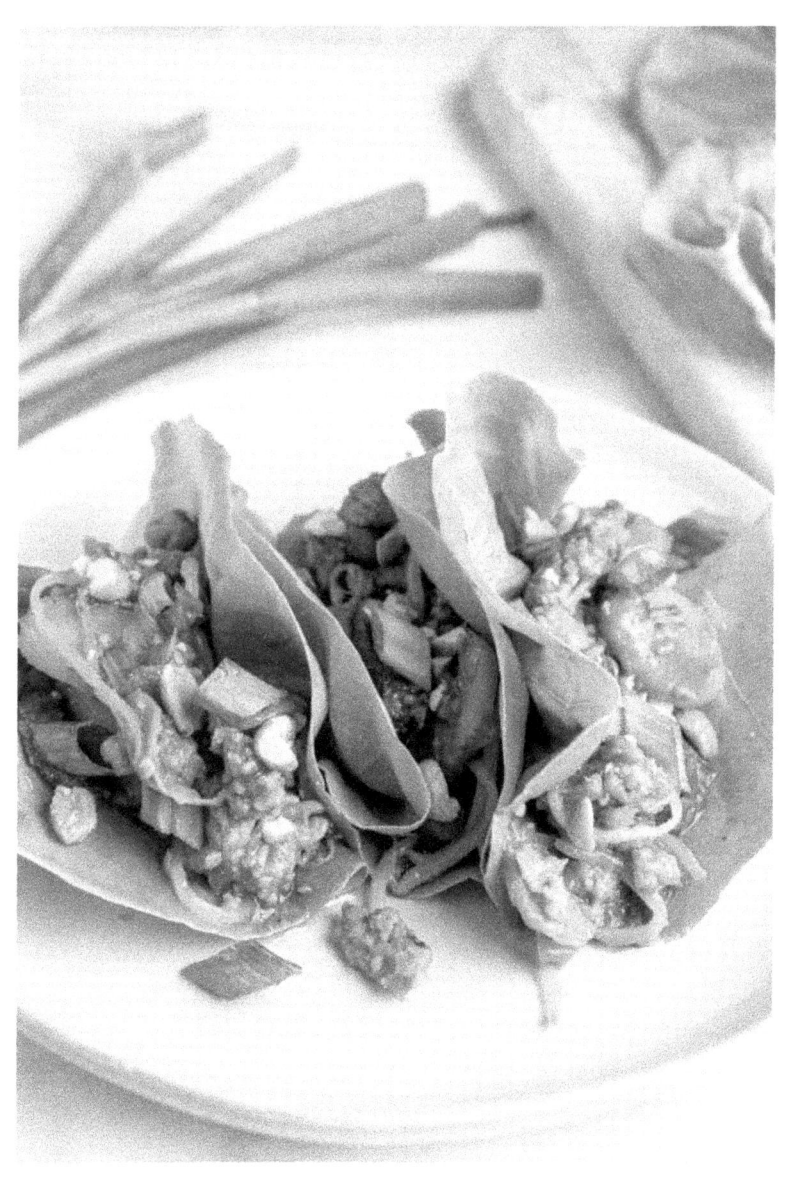

Balsamic Chicken and Vegetables

Serving: 2

Prep Time: 15 minutes

Cook Time: 25 minutes

Ingredients:

4 chicken thigh, boneless and skinless

5 stalks of asparagus, halved

1 pepper, cut in chunks

1/2 red onion, diced

½ cup carrots, sliced

1 garlic clove, minced

2-ounces mushrooms, diced

¼ cup balsamic vinegar

1 tablespoon olive oil

½ teaspoon stevia

½ tablespoon oregano

Sunflower seeds and pepper as needed

How To:

1. Pre-heat your oven to 425 degrees F.

2. Take a bowl and add all of the vegetables and blend.

3. Add spices and oil and blend.

4. Dip the chicken pieces into spice mix and coat them well.

5. Place the veggies and chicken onto a pan during a single layer.

6. Cook for 25 minutes.

7. Serve and enjoy!

Nutrition (Per Serving)

Calories: 401

Fat: 17g

Net Carbohydrates: 11g

Protein: 48g

Cream Dredged Corn Platter

Serving: 3

Prep Time: 10 minutes

Cook Time: 4 hours

Ingredients:

3 cups corn

2 ounces cream cheese, cubed

2 tablespoons milk

2 tablespoons whipping cream

2 tablespoons butter, melted

Salt and pepper as needed

1 tablespoon green onion, chopped

How To:

1. Add corn, cheese, milk, light whipping cream, butter, salt and pepper to your Slow Cooker.

2. provides it a pleasant toss to combine everything well.

3. Place lid and cook on LOW for 4 hours.

4. Divide the combination amongst serving platters.

5. Serve and enjoy!

Nutrition (Per Serving)

Calories: 261

Fat: 11g

Carbohydrates: 17g

Protein: 6g

Exuberant Sweet Potatoes

Serving: 4

Prep Time: 5 minutes

Cook Time: 7-8 hours

Ingredients:

6 sweet potatoes, washed and dried

How To:

1. Loosely botch 7-8 pieces of aluminium foil within the bottom of your Slow Cooker, covering about half the area.
2. Prick each potato 6-8 times employing a fork.
3. Wrap each potato with foil and seal them.
4. Place wrapped potatoes within the cooker on top of the foil bed.
5. Place lid and cook on LOW for 7-8 hours.
6. Use tongs to get rid of the potatoes and unwrap them.
7. Serve and enjoy!

Nutrition (Per Serving)

Calories: 129

Fat: 0g

Carbohydrates: 30g

Protein: 2g

Leek and Cauliflower Soup

Serving: 6

Prep Time: 10 minutes

Cook Time: 40 minutes

Ingredients:

3 cups cauliflower, riced

1 bay leaf

1 teaspoon herbs de Provence

2 garlic cloves, peeled and diced

½ cup coconut milk

2 ½ cups vegetable stock

1 tablespoon coconut oil

½ teaspoon cracked pepper

1 leek, chopped

How To:

1. Take a pot, heat oil into it.

2. Sauté the leeks in the oil for 5 minutes.

3. Add the garlic and then stir-cook for another minute.

4. Add all the remaining ingredients and mix them well.

5. Cook for 30 minutes.

6. Stir occasionally.

7. Blend the soup until smooth by using an immersion blender.

8. Serve hot and enjoy!

Nutrition (Per Serving)

Calories: 90

Fat: 7g

Carbohydrates: 4g

Protein: 2g

Dreamy Zucchini Bowl

Serving: 4

Prep Time: 10 minutes

Cook Time: 20 minutes

Ingredients:

1 onion, chopped

3 zucchini, cut into medium chunks

2 tablespoons coconut almond milk

2 garlic cloves, minced

4 cups vegetable stock

2 tablespoons coconut oil

Pinch of sunflower seeds

Black pepper to taste

How To:

1. Take a pot and place it over medium heat.
2. Add oil and let it heat up.

3. Add zucchini, garlic, onion and stir.
4. Cook for 5 minutes.
5. Add stock, sunflower seeds, pepper and stir.
6. Bring to a boil and reduce heat.
7. Simmer for 20 minutes.
8. Remove from heat and add coconut almond milk.
9. Use an immersion blender until smooth.
10. Ladle into soup bowls and serve.
11. Enjoy!

Nutrition (Per Serving)

Calories: 160

Fat: 2g

Carbohydrates: 4g

Protein: 7g

Cold Crab and Watermelon Soup

Serving: 4

Prep Time: 10 minutes + chill time

Cook Time: nil

Ingredients:

¼ cup basil, chopped

2 pounds tomatoes

5 cups watermelon, cubed

¼ cup wine vinegar

2 garlic cloves, minced

1 zucchini, chopped

Pepper to taste

1 cup crabmeat

How To:

1. Take your blender and add tomatoes, basil, vinegar, 4 cups watermelon, garlic, 1/3 cup oil, pepper and pulse well.

2. Transfer to fridge and chill for 1 hour.

3. Divide into bowls and add zucchini, crab and remaining watermelon.

4. Serve and enjoy!

Nutrition (Per Serving)

Calories: 121

Fat: 3g

Carbohydrates: 4g

Protein: 8g

Paleo Lemon and Garlic Soup

Serving: 4

Prep Time: 10 minutes

Cook Time: 10 minutes

Ingredients:

6 cups shellfish stock

1 tablespoon garlic, minced

1 tablespoon coconut oil, melted

2 whole eggs

½ cup lemon juice

Pinch of salt

White pepper to taste

1 tablespoon arrowroot powder

Finely chopped cilantro for serving

How To:

1. Heat up a pot with oil over medium high heat.

2. Add garlic, stir cook for 2 minutes.

3. Add stock (reserve ½ cup for later use).

4. Stir and bring mix to a simmer.

5. Take a bowl and add eggs, sea salt, pepper, reserved stock, lemon juice and arrowroot.

6. Whisk well.

7. Pour in to the soup and cook for a few minutes.

8. Ladle soup into bowls and serve with chopped cilantro.

9. Enjoy!

Nutrition (Per Serving)

Calories: 135

Fat: 3g

Carbohydrates: 12g

Protein: 8

Brussels Soup

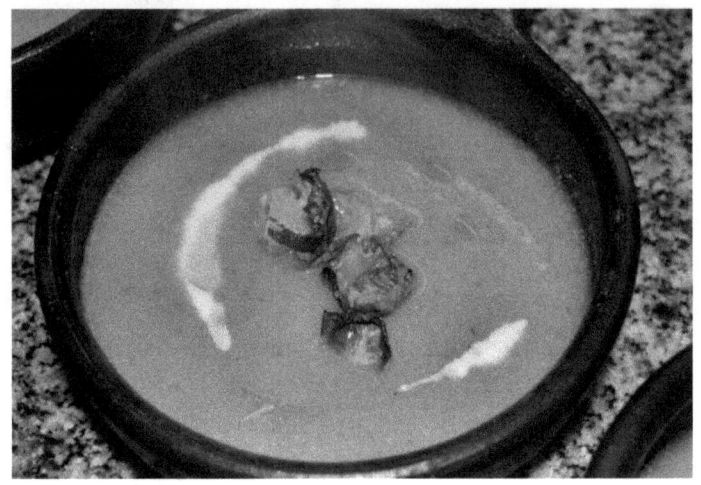

Serving: 4

Prep Time: 10 minutes

Cook Time: 20 minutes

Ingredients:

2 tablespoons olive oil

1 yellow onion, chopped

2 pounds Brussels sprouts, trimmed and halved

4 cups chicken stock

¼ cup coconut cream

How To:

1. Take a pot and place it over medium heat.
2. Add oil and let it heat up.
3. Add onion and stir-cook for 3 minutes.
4. Add Brussels sprouts and stir, cook for 2 minutes.
5. Add stock and black pepper, stir and bring to a simmer.
6. Cook for 20 minutes more.
7. Use an immersion blender to make the soup creamy.
8. Add coconut cream and stir well.
9. Ladle into soup bowls and serve.
10. Enjoy!

Nutrition (Per Serving)

Calories: 200

Fat: 11g

Carbohydrates: 6g

Protein: 11g

Spring Soup and Poached Egg

Serving: 4

Prep Time: 5 minutes

Cook Time: 15 minutes

Ingredients:

2 whole eggs

32 ounces chicken broth

1 head romaine lettuce, chopped

How To:

1. Bring the chicken broth to a boil.

2. Reduce the heat and poach the 2 eggs in the broth for 5 minutes.

3. Take two bowls and transfer the eggs into a separate bowl.

4. Add chopped romaine lettuce into the broth and cook for a few minutes.

5. Serve the broth with lettuce into the bowls.

6. Enjoy!

Nutrition (Per Serving)

Calories: 150

Fat: 5g

Carbohydrates: 6g

Protein: 16g

Lobster Bisque

Serving: 4

Prep Time: 10 minutes

Cook Time: 15 minutes

Ingredients:

¾ pound lobster, cooked and lobster

4 cups chicken broth

2 garlic cloves, chopped

¼ teaspoon pepper

½ teaspoon paprika

1 yellow onion, chopped

½ teaspoon salt

14 ½ ounces tomatoes, diced

1 tablespoon coconut oil

1 cup low fat cream

How To:

1. Take a stockpot and add the coconut oil over medium heat.

2. Then sauté the garlic and onion for 3 to 5 minutes.

3. Add diced tomatoes, spices and chicken broth and bring to a boil.

4. Reduce to a simmer, then simmer for about 10 minutes.

5. Add the warmed heavy cream to the soup.

6. Blend the soup till creamy by using an immersion blender.

7. Stir in cooked lobster.

8. Serve and enjoy!

Nutrition (Per Serving)

Calories: 180

Fat: 11g

Carbohydrates: 6g

Protein: 16g

Tomato Bisque

Serving: 4

Prep Time: 10 minutes

Cook Time: 40 minutes

Ingredients:

4 cups chicken broth

1 cup low fat cream

1 teaspoon thyme dried

3 cups canned whole, peeled tomatoes

2 tablespoons almond butter

3 garlic cloves, peeled

Pepper as needed

How To:

1. Take a stockpot and first add the butter to the bottom of a stockpot.

2. Then add all the ingredients except heavy cream into it.

3. Bring to a boil.

4. Simmer for 40 minutes.

5. Warm the heavy cream and stir into the soup.

6. Serve and enjoy!

Nutrition (Per Serving)

Calories: 141

Fat: 12g

Carbohydrates: 4g

Protein: 4g

Chipotle Chicken Chowder

Serving: 4

Prep Time: 10 minutes

Cook Time: 23 minutes

Ingredients:

1 medium onion, chopped

2 garlic cloves, minced

6 bacon slices, chopped

4 cups jicama, cubed

3 cups chicken stock

1 teaspoon salt

2 cups low-fat, cream1 tablespoon olive oil

2 tablespoons fresh cilantro, chopped

1 ¼ pounds chicken, thigh boneless, cut into 1 inch chunks ½ teaspoon pepper

1 chipotle pepper, minced

How To:

1. Heat olive oil over medium heat in a large sized saucepan, add bacon.

2. Cook until crispy, add onion, garlic, and jicama.

3. Cook for 7 minutes, add chicken stock and chicken.

4. Bring to a boil and reduce temperature to low.

5. Simmer for 10 minutes

6. Season with salt and pepper.

7. Add heavy cream and chipotle, simmer for 5 minutes.

8. Sprinkle chopped cilantro and serve, enjoy!

Nutrition (Per Serving)

Calories: 350

Fat: 22g

Carbohydrates: 8g

Protein: 22g

Cinnamon Salmon

Serving: 4

Prep Time: 10 minutes

Cook Time: 10 minutes

Ingredients:

2 salmon fillets, boneless and skin on

Pepper to taste

1 tablespoon cinnamon powder

1 tablespoon organic olive oil

How To:

1. Take a pan and place it over medium heat, add oil and let it heat up.
2. Add pepper, cinnamon and stir.
3. Add salmon, skin side up and cook for five minutes on each side.
4. Divide between plates and serve.
5. Enjoy!

Nutrition (Per Serving)

Calories: 220

Fat: 8g

Carbohydrates: 11g

Protein: 8g

Scallop and Strawberry Mix

Serving: 4

Prep Time: 10 minutes

Cook Time: 6 minutes

Ingredients:

ounces scallops

½ cup Pico De Gallo

½ cup strawberries, chopped

1 tablespoon lime juice

Pepper to taste

How To:

1. Take a pan and place it over medium heat, add scallops and cook for 3 minutes on each side.

2. Remove heat.

3. Take a bowl and add strawberries, juice , Pico De Gallo, scallops, pepper and toss well.

4. Serve and enjoy!

Nutrition (Per Serving)

Calories: 169

Fat: 2g

Carbohydrates: 8g

Protein: 13g

Salmon and Orange Dish

Serving: 4

Prep Time: 10 minutes

Cook Time: 15 minutes

Ingredients:

salmon fillets

cup orange juice

tablespoons arrowroot and water mixture 1 teaspoon orange peel, grated 1 teaspoon black pepper

How To:

1. Add the listed ingredients to your pot.
2. Lock the lid and cook on high for 12 minutes.
3. Release the pressure naturally.
4. Serve and enjoy!

Nutrition (Per Serving)

Calories:583

Fat: 20g

Carbohydrates: 71g

Protein: 33g

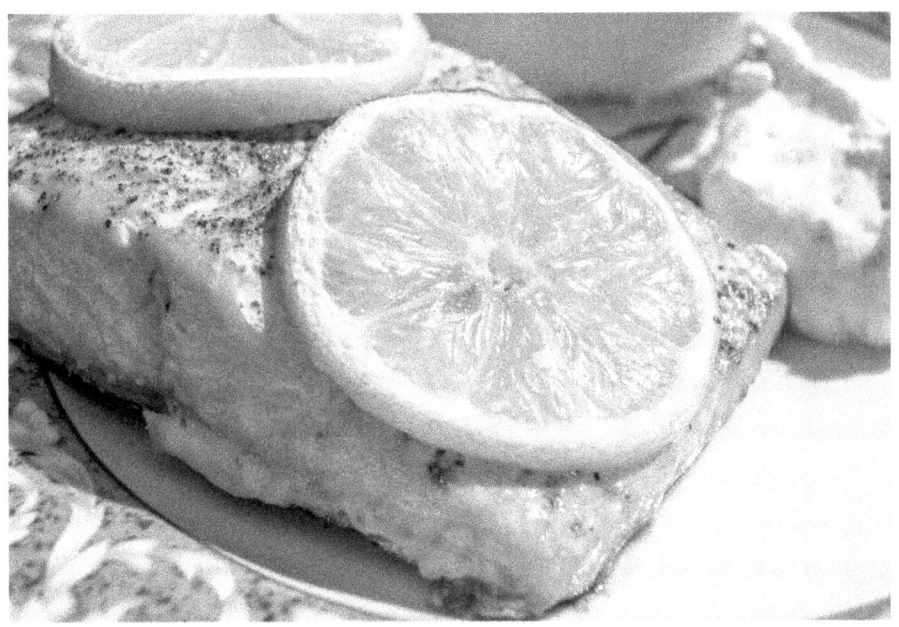

Mesmerizing Coconut Haddock

Serving: 3

Prep Time: 10 minutes

Cook Time: 12 minutes

Ingredients:

Haddock fillets, 5 ounces each, boneless 2 tablespoons coconut oil, melted

1 cup coconut, shredded and unsweetened

¼ cup hazelnuts, ground Sunflower seeds to taste

How To:

1. Pre-heat your oven to 400 degrees F.
2. Line a baking sheet with parchment paper.
3. Keep it on the side.
4. Pat fish fillets with towel and season with sunflower seeds.
5. Take a bowl and stir in hazelnuts and shredded coconut.

6. Drag fish fillets through the coconut mix until each side are coated well.

7. Transfer to baking dish.

8. Brush with copra oil .

9. Bake for about 12 minutes until flaky.

10. Serve and enjoy!

Nutrition (Per Serving)

Calories: 299

Fat: 24g

Carbohydrates: 1g

Protein: 20g

Asparagus and Lemon Salmon Dish

Serving: 3

Prep Time: 5 minutes

Cook Time: 15 minutes

Ingredients:

2 salmon fillets, 6 ounces each, skin on Sunflower seeds to taste

1-pound asparagus, trimmed 2 cloves garlic, minced tablespoons almond butter ¼ cup cashew cheese

How To:

Pre-heat your oven to 400 degrees F.

Line a baking sheet with oil.

Take a kitchen towel and pat your salmon dry, season as needed.

1. Put salmon onto the baking sheet and arrange asparagus around it.

2. Place a pan over medium heat and melt almond butter.

3. Add garlic and cook for 3 minutes until garlic browns slightly.

4. Drizzle sauce over salmon.

5. Sprinkle salmon with cheese and bake for 12 minutes until salmon looks cooked all the way and is flaky.

6. Serve and enjoy!

Nutrition (Per Serving)

Calories: 434

Fat: 26g

Carbohydrates: 6g

Protein: 42g

Lamb Curry with Tomatoes And Spinach

Prep time: 10 minutes

Cook time: 12 minutes

Servings: 4

Ingredients

Olive oil – 1 tsp

Lean boneless lamb – 1 pound, sliced thinly Onion – 1, chopped

Garlic – 3 cloves, minced Red bell pepper – 1, chopped Salt-free tomato paste – 2 Tbsp.

Salt-free curry powder – 1 Tbsp.

No-salt-added diced tomatoes – 1(15-ounce) can

Fresh baby spinach – 10 ounces

Low-sodium beef or vegetable broth - ½ cup

Red wine – ¼ cup

Chopped fresh cilantro – ¼ cup Ground black pepper to taste

Method

1. Heat the oil in a pan.

2. Add lamb and brown both sides, about 2 minutes.

3. Add garlic, onion, and bell pepper. Stir-fry for 2 minutes. Stir in the curry powder and tomato paste.

4. Add the tomatoes with juice, spinach, broth, and wine and stir to mix.

5. Stir-fry for 3 to 4 minutes and lamb has cooked through.

6. Remove from heat. Season with pepper and stir in cilantro.

7. Serve.

Nutritional Facts Per Serving

Calories: 238

Fat: 7g

Carb: 14g

Protein: 27g

Sodium 167mg

Pomegranate-Marinated Leg of Lamb

Prep time: 10 minutes

Cook time: 20 minutes

Servings: 6

Ingredients

For the marinate

Bottled pomegranate juice - ½ cup

Hearty red wine – ½ cup

Ground cumin - 1 tsp.

Dried oregano – 1 tsp.

Crushed hot red pepper – ½ tsp.

Garlic – 3 cloves, minced

For the lamb

Boneless leg of lamb – 1 ¾ pound, butterflied and fat trimmed

Kosher salt – ½ tsp.

Olive oil spray

Method

1. To make the marinade, whisk everything in a bowl and transfer to a zippered plastic bag.

2. To prepare the lamb: add the lamb to the bag, press out the air, and close the bag. Marinate for 1 hour in the refrigerator.

3. Preheat the broiler (8 inches from the source of heat).

4. Remove the lamb from the marinade, blot with paper towels, but do not dry completely.

5. Season with salt. Spray the broiler rack with oil.

6. Place the lamb on the rack and broil, turning occasionally, about 20 minutes, or until lamb is browned and reaches 130F.

7. Remove from heat, slice and serve with carving juices on top.

Nutritional Facts Per Serving

Calories: 273

Fat: 15g

Carb: 0g

Protein: 31g

Sodium 219mg

Beef Fajitas with Peppers

Prep time: 10 minutes

Cook time: 12 minutes

Servings: 6

Ingredients

Olive oil – 2 tsp. plus more for the spray

Sirloin steak – 1 pound, cut into bite-size pieces

Red bell pepper – 1, chopped

Green bell pepper – 1, chopped

Red onion – 1, chopped

Garlic - 2 cloves, minced

DASH friendly Mexican seasoning – 1 Tbsp. (or any seasoning without salt)

Boston lettuce leaves – 12 for serving Lime wedges or corn tortillas for serving

Method

Heat oil in a skillet.

Add half of the sirloin and cook until browned on both sides, about 2 minutes. Transfer to a plate.

Then repeat with the remaining sirloin.

Heat the 2 tsp. oil in the skillet.

Add onion, bell peppers, and garlic, cook and stir for 7 minutes or until tender.

Stir in the beef with any juices and the seasoning. Transfer to a plate.

Fill lettuce lead with beef mixture and drizzle lime juice on top.

Roll up and serve.

Nutritional Facts Per Serving

Calories: 231

Fat: 12g

Carb: 6g

Protein: 24g

Sodium 59mg

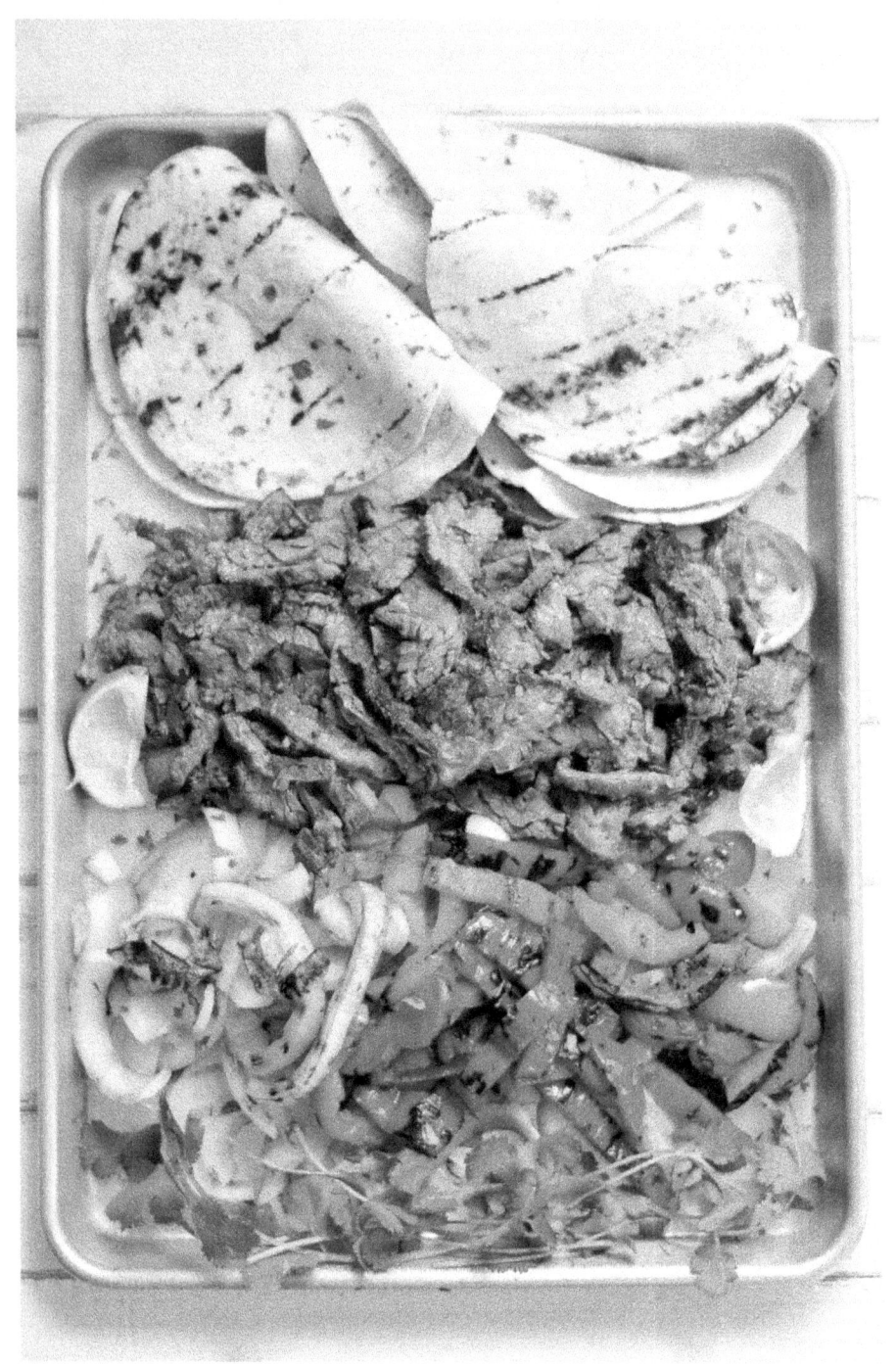

Pork Medallions with Herbs De Provence

Prep time: 5 minutes

Cook time: 10 minutes

Servings: 2

Ingredients

Pork tenderloin – 8 ounces, cut into 6 pieces (crosswise)

Ground black pepper to taste Herbs de Provence – ½ tsp. Dry white wine – ¼ cup

Method

1. Season the pork with black pepper.

2. Place the pork between waxed paper sheets and roll with a rolling pin until about ¼ inch thick.

3. Cook the pork in a pan for 2 to 3 minutes on each side.

4. Remove from heat and season with the herb.

5. Place the pork on plates and keep warm.

6. Cook the wine in the pan until boiling. Scrape to get the brown bits from the bottom.

7.   Serve pork with the sauce.

Nutritional Facts Per Serving

Calories: 120

Fat: 2g

Carb: 1g

Protein: 24g

Sodium 62mg

Ravaging Blueberry Muffin

Serving: 4

Prep Time: 10 minutes

Cook Time: 30 minutes

Ingredients:

1 cup almond flour

Pinch of sunflower seeds

1/8 teaspoon baking soda

1 whole egg

2 tablespoons coconut oil, melted

½ cup coconut almond milk

¼ cup fresh blueberries

How To:

1. Pre-heat your oven to 350 degrees F.
2. Line a muffin tin with paper muffin cups.

3. Add almond flour, sunflower seeds, baking soda to a bowl and mix, keep it on the side.

4. Take another bowl and add egg, coconut oil, coconut almond milk and mix.

5. Add mix to flour mix and gently combine until incorporated.

6. Mix in blueberries and fill the cupcakes tins with batter.

7. Bake for 20-25 minutes.

8. Enjoy!

Nutrition (Per Serving)

Calories: 167

Fat: 15g

Carbohydrates: 2.1g

Protein: 5.2g

The Coconut Loaf

Serving: 4

Prep Time: 15 minutes

Cook Time: 40 minutes

Ingredients:

1 ½ tablespoons coconut flour

¼ teaspoon baking powder

1/8 teaspoon sunflower seeds

1 tablespoons coconut oil, melted

1 whole egg

How To:

1. Pre-heat your oven to 350 degrees F.
2. Add coconut flour, baking powder, sunflower seeds.
3. Add coconut oil, eggs and stir well until mixed.
4. Leave batter for several minutes.
5. Pour half batter onto baking pan.

6. Spread it to form a circle, repeat with remaining batter.

7. Bake in oven for 10 minutes.

8. Once you have a golden-brown texture, let it cool and serve.

9. Enjoy!

Nutrition (Per Serving)

Calories: 297

Fat: 14g

Carbohydrates: 15g

Protein: 15g

Fresh Figs with Walnuts and Ricotta

Serving: 4

Prep Time: 5 minutes

Cook Time: 2-3 minutes

Ingredients:

8 dried figs, halved

¼ cup ricotta cheese

16 walnuts, halved

1 tablespoon honey

How To:

1. Take a skillet and place it over medium heat, add walnuts and toast for 2 minutes.

2. Top figs with cheese and walnuts.

3. Drizzle honey on top.

4. Enjoy!

Nutrition (Per Serving)

Calories: 142

Fat: 8g

Carbohydrates:10g

Protein:4g

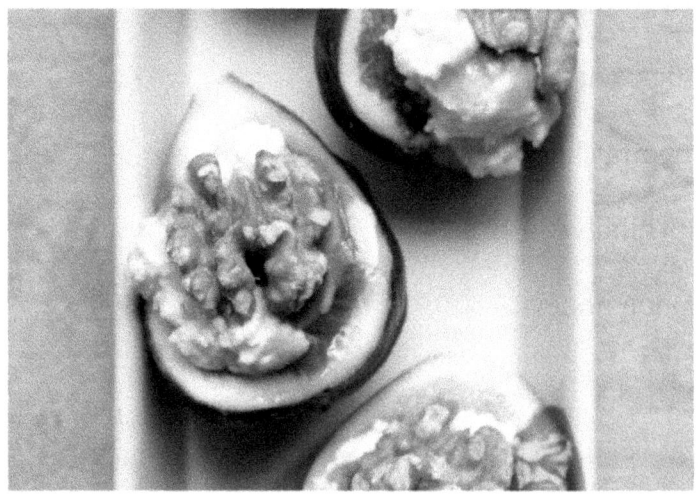

Authentic Medjool Date Truffles

Serving: 4

Prep Time: 10-15 minutes

Cook Time: Nil

Ingredients:

2 tablespoons peanut oil

½ cup popcorn kernels

1/3 cup peanuts, chopped

1/3 cup peanut almond butter

¼ cup wildflower honey

How To:

1. Take a pot and add popcorn kernels, peanut oil.

2. Place it over medium heat and shake the pot gently until all corn has popped.

3. Take a saucepan and add honey, gently simmer for 2-3 minutes.

4. Add peanut almond butter and stir.

5. Coat popcorn with the mixture and enjoy!

Nutrition (Per Serving)

Calories: 430

Fat: 20g

Carbohydrates: 56g

Protein 9g

Tasty Mediterranean Peanut Almond butter Popcorns

Serving: 4

Prep Time: 5 minutes + 20 minutes chill time

Cook Time: 2-3 minutes

Ingredients:

3 cups Medjool dates, chopped

12 ounces brewed coffee 1 cup pecans, chopped ½ cup coconut, shredded ½ cup cocoa powder

How To:

1. Soak dates in warm coffee for 5 minutes.

2. Remove dates from coffee and mash them, making a fine smooth mixture.

3. Stir in remaining ingredients (except cocoa powder) and form small balls out of the mixture.

4. Coat with cocoa powder, serve and enjoy!

Nutrition (Per Serving)

Calories: 265

Fat: 12g

Carbohydrates: 43g

Protein 3g

Just A Minute Worth Muffin

Serving: 2

Prep Time: 5 minutes

Cooking Time: 1 minute

Ingredients:

Coconut oil for grease

2 teaspoons coconut flour

1 pinch baking soda

1 pinch sunflower seed

1 whole egg

How To:

1. Grease ramekin dish with coconut oil and keep it on the side.

2. Add ingredients to a bowl and combine until no lumps.

3. Pour batter into ramekin.

4. Microwave for 1 minute on HIGH.

5. Slice in half and serve.

6. Enjoy!

Nutrition (Per Serving)

Total Carbs: 5.4

Fiber: 2g

Protein: 7.3g

Hearty Almond Bread

Serving: 8

Prep Time: 15 minutes

Cook Time: 60 minutes

Ingredients:

3 cups almond flour

1 teaspoon baking soda

2 teaspoons baking powder

¼ teaspoon sunflower seeds

¼ cup almond milk

½ cup + 2 tablespoons olive oil

3 whole eggs

How To:

1. Pre-heat your oven to 300 degrees F.
2. Take a 9x5 inch loaf pan and grease, keep it on the side.

3. Add listed ingredients to a bowl and pour the batter into the loaf pan.

4. Bake for 60 minutes.

5. Once baked, remove from oven and let it cool.

6. Slice and serve!

Nutrition (Per Serving)

Calories: 277

Fat: 21g

Carbohydrates: 7g

Protein: 10g

Refreshing Mango and Pear Smoothie

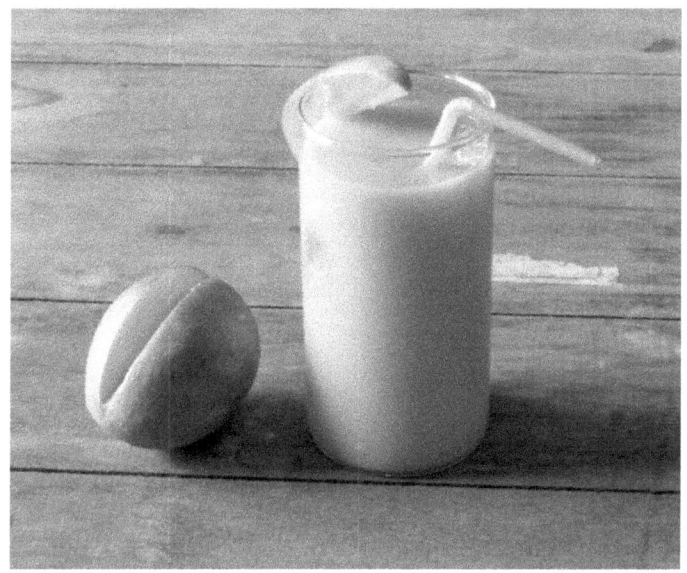

Serving: 1

Prep Time: 10 minutes

Cook Time: Nil

Ingredients:

1 ripe mango, cored and chopped

½ mango, peeled, pitted and chopped

1 cup kale, chopped

½ cup plain Greek yogurt

2 ice cubes

How To:

1. Add pear, mango, yogurt, kale, and mango to a blender and puree.

2. Add ice and blend until you have a smooth texture.

3. Serve and enjoy!

Nutrition (Per Serving)

Calories: 293

Fat: 8g

Carbohydrates: 53g

Protein: 8g

Coconut and Hazelnut Chilled Glass

Serving: 1

Prep Time: 10 minutes

Ingredients:

½ cup coconut almond milk

¼ cup hazelnuts, chopped

1 ½ cups water

1 pack stevia

How To:

1. Add listed ingredients to blender.
2. Blend until you have a smooth and creamy texture.
3. Serve chilled and enjoy!

Nutrition (Per Serving)

Calories: 457

Fat: 46g

Carbohydrates: 12g

Protein: 7g

The Mocha Shake

Serving: 1

Prep Time: 10 minutes

Ingredients:

1 cup whole almond milk

2 tablespoons cocoa powder2 packs stevia

1 cup brewed coffee, chilled

1 tablespoon coconut oil

How To:

1. Add listed ingredients to blender.
2. Blend until you have a smooth and creamy texture.
3. Serve chilled and enjoy!

Nutrition (Per Serving)

Calories: 293

Fat: 23g

Carbohydrates: 19g

Protein: 10g

Cinnamon Chiller

Serving: 1

Prep Time: 10 minutes

Ingredients:

1 cup unsweetened almond milk

2 tablespoons vanilla protein powder

½ teaspoon cinnamon

¼ teaspoon vanilla extract

1 tablespoon chia seeds

1 cup ice cubs

How To:

1. Add listed ingredients to blender.
2. Blend until you have a smooth and creamy texture.
3. Serve chilled and enjoy!

Nutrition (Per Serving)

Calories: 145

Fat: 4g

Carbohydrates: 1.6g

Protein: 0.6g

Hearty Alkaline Strawberry Summer Deluxe

Serving: 2

Prep Time: 5 minutes

Ingredients:

½ cup organic strawberries/blueberries

Half a banana

2 cups coconut water ½ inch ginger

Juice of 2 grapefruits

How To:

1. Add all the listed ingredients to your blender.
2. Blend until smooth.
3. Add a few ice cubes and serve the smoothie.
4. Enjoy!

Nutrition (Per Serving)

Calories: 200

Fat: 10g

Carbohydrates: 14g

Protein 2g

Mesmerizing Brussels and Pistachios

Serving: 4

Prep Time: 15 minutes

Cook Time: 15 minutes

Ingredients:

1-pound Brussels sprouts, tough bottom trimmed and halved lengthwise

1 tablespoon extra-virgin olive oil

Sunflower seeds and pepper as needed

½ cup roasted pistachios, chopped Juice of ½ lemon

How To:

1. Pre-heat your oven to 400 degrees F.

2. Line a baking sheet with aluminum foil and keep it on the side.

3. Take a large bowl and add Brussels sprouts with olive oil and coat well.

4. Season sea sunflower seeds, pepper, spread veggies evenly on sheet.

5. Bake for 15 minutes until lightly caramelized.

6. Remove from oven and transfer to a serving bowl.

7. Toss with pistachios and lemon juice.

8. Serve warm and enjoy!

Nutrition (Per Serving)

Calories: 126

Fat: 7g

Carbohydrates: 14g

Protein: 6g

Brussels's Fever

Serving: 4

Prep Time: 10 minutes

Cook Time: 20 minutes

Ingredients:

2 tablespoons olive oil

1 yellow onion, chopped

2 pounds Brussels sprouts, trimmed and halved

4 cups vegetable stock

¼ cup coconut cream

How To:

1. Take a pot and place it over medium heat.
2. Add oil and let it heat up.
3. Add onion and stir-cook for 3 minutes.
4. Add Brussels sprouts and stir, cook for 2 minutes.
5. Add stock and black pepper, stir and bring to a simmer.

6. Cook for 20 minutes more.
7. Use an immersion blender to make the soup creamy.
8. Add coconut cream and stir well.
9. Ladle into soup bowls and serve.
10. Enjoy!

Nutrition (Per Serving)

Calories: 200

Fat: 11g

Carbohydrates: 6g

Protein: 11g

Hearty Garlic and Kale Platter

Serving: 4

Prep Time: 5 minutes

Cook Time: 10 minutes

Ingredients:

1 bunch kale

2 tablespoons olive oil

4 garlic cloves, minced

How To:

1. Carefully tear the kale into bite sized portions, making sure to remove the stem.
2. Discard the stems.
3. Take a large sized pot and place it over medium heat.
4. Add olive oil and let the oil heat up.
5. Add garlic and stir for 2 minutes.
6. Add kale and cook for 5-10 minutes.

7. Serve!

Nutrition (Per Serving)

Calories: 121

Fat: 8g

Carbohydrates: 5g

Protein: 4g

Acorn Squash with Mango Chutney

Serving: 4

Prep Time: 10 minutes

Cook Time: 3 hours 10 minutes

Ingredients:

1 large acorn squash

¼ cup mango chutney

¼ cup flaked coconut

Salt and pepper as needed

How To:

1. Cut the squash into quarters and remove the seeds, discard the pulp.

2. Spray your cooker with olive oil.

3. Transfer the squash to the Slow Cooker and place lid.

4. Take a bowl and add coconut and chutney, mix well and divide the mixture into the center of the Squash.

5. Season well.

6. Place lid on top and cook on LOW for 2-3 hours.

7. Enjoy!

Nutrition (Per Serving)

Calories: 226

Fat: 6g

Carbohydrates: 24g

Protein: 17g

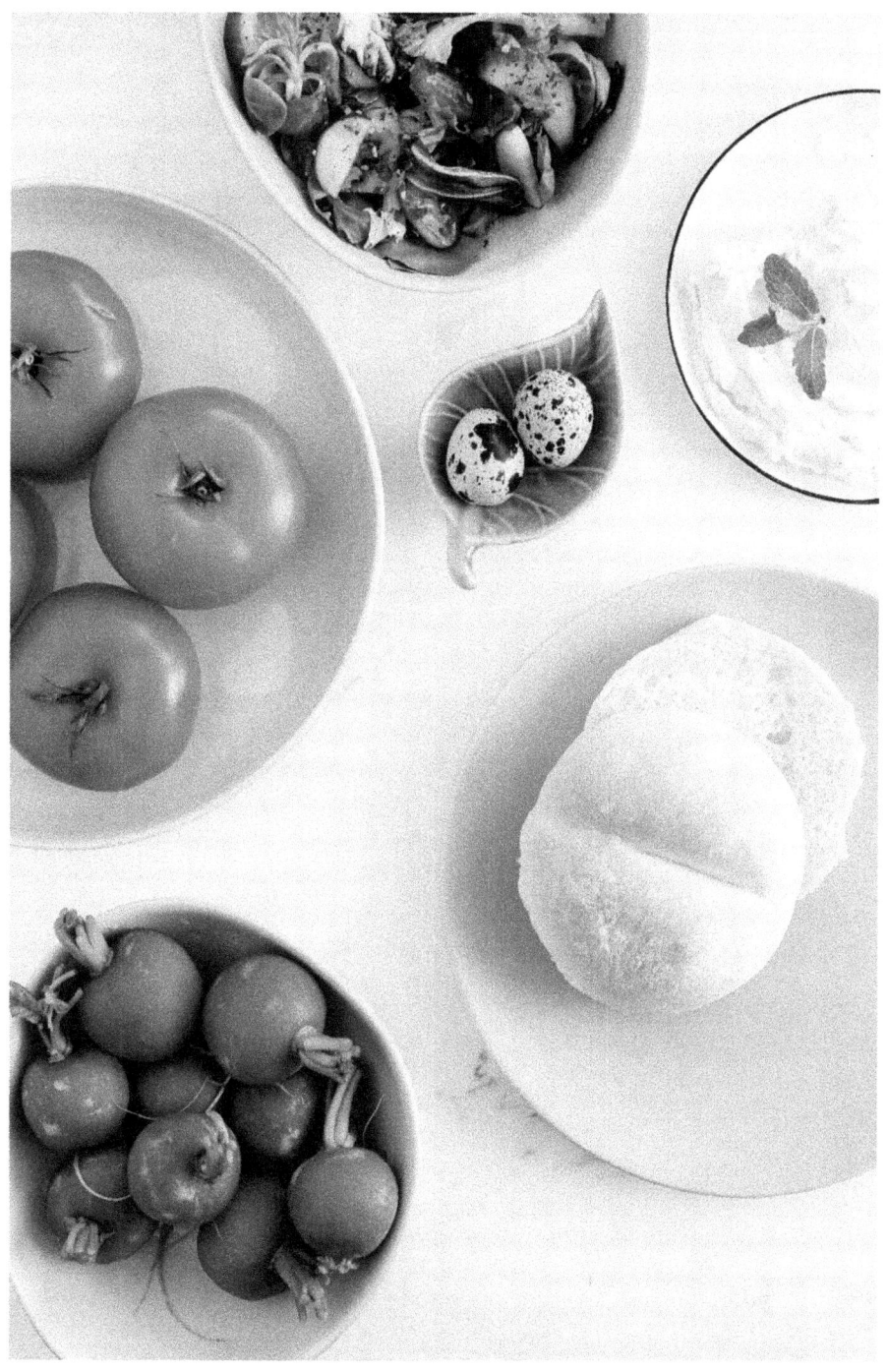

www.ingramcontent.com/pod-product-compliance
Lightning Source LLC
Chambersburg PA
CBHW071112030426
42336CB00013BA/2050